THE EFFECTIVE WEIGHT LOSS COOKBOOK

Your Guide to Flavorful and Effective Weight Loss Cooking

MADIE MERTZ

Copyright © 2024 Madie Mertz.

All rights reserved. No part of this book may be reproduced, distributed, or transmitted in any form or by any means, including photocopying, recording, or other electronic or mechanical methods, without the prior written permission of the publisher, except in the case of brief quotations embodied in critical reviews and certain other noncommercial uses permitted by copyright law.

ABOUT THE AUTHOR

Madie Mertz is a passionate advocate for healthy living and culinary exploration. With a background in nutrition and a love for creating delicious, wholesome meals, Madie is dedicated to helping others achieve their health and wellness goals through balanced eating and mindful living.

As a certified nutritionist and avid home cook, Madie understands the importance of nourishing the body with nutrient-dense foods that support overall well-being. Her approach to cooking emphasizes simplicity, flavor, and the joy of sharing nutritious meals with family and friends.

Through "The Effective Weight Loss Cookbook," Madie shares her expertise and passion, offering a collection of recipes and strategies designed to make weight loss enjoyable and sustainable. Whether you're embarking on a new health journey or looking to maintain your current lifestyle, Madie's recipes provide delicious options that align with your goals.

Table of Contents

About the Author 4

Introduction 10

Chapter 1 13

   Introduction to Effective Weight Loss 13

   recipes 15

      1. Grilled Chicken with Quinoa and Veggies 15

      2. Baked Salmon with Asparagus 16

      3. Turkey and Vegetable Stir-Fry 17

      4. Veggie-Packed Cauliflower Rice Bowl 18

      5. Spaghetti Squash with Tomato Basil Sauce 19

      6. Chicken and Avocado Salad 20

Chapter 2 23

   Energizing Breakfasts 23

   recipes 23

      1. Avocado Toast with Poached Egg 23

      2. Greek Yogurt Parfait 24

      3. Spinach and Feta Omelette 25

      4. Berry and Banana Smoothie Bowl 26

      5. Quinoa Breakfast Bowl 27

      6. Veggie-Packed Breakfast Burrito 28

Chapter 3 31

Satisfying Lunches 31

recipes 31

    1. Quinoa and Black Bean Salad 31

    2. Turkey and Avocado Lettuce Wraps 32

    3. Grilled Chicken and Veggie Skewers 34

    4. Cauliflower Fried Rice 35

    5. Lentil and Spinach Soup 36

    6. Greek Yogurt Chicken Salad 37

Chapter 4 39

Delicious Dinners 39

recipes 39

    1. Lemon Herb Grilled Chicken 39

    2. Quinoa Stuffed Bell Peppers 40

    3. Baked Salmon with Asparagus 41

    4. Spaghetti Squash with Turkey Marinara 42

    5. Cauliflower Fried Rice 44

    6. Zucchini Noodles with Pesto and Grilled Shrimp 45

Chapter 5 47

Smart Snacks and Appetizers 47

recipes 47

    1. Cucumber Hummus Bites 47

- 2. Greek Yogurt and Berry Parfait 48
- 3. Avocado and Black Bean Salsa 49
- 4. Baked Zucchini Chips 50
- 5. Spicy Roasted Chickpeas 51
- 6. Stuffed Mini Bell Peppers 52

Chapter 6 55
- Guilt-Free Desserts 55
- recipes 55
  - 1. Chocolate Avocado Mousse 55
  - 2. Greek Yogurt Berry Parfait 56
  - 3. Baked Apples with Cinnamon 57
  - 4. Chia Seed Pudding 58
  - 5. Banana Oat Cookies 59
  - 6. Lemon Yogurt Cake 59

Chapter 7 63
- Smoothies and Beverages 63
- Recipes 63
  - 1. Green Detox Smoothie 63
  - 2. Berry Protein Smoothie 64
  - 3. Tropical Mango Smoothie 65
  - 4. Matcha Green Tea Latte 65
  - 5. Cucumber Mint Detox Water 66

6. Golden Milk 67

Chapter 8 69

   Meal Planning and Prep 69

   Tips for Effective Meal Planning and Prep 69

   RECIPES 70

     1. Grilled Lemon Herb Chicken 70

     2. Quinoa and Black Bean Salad 71

     3. Baked Salmon with Asparagus 72

     4. Turkey Meatballs with Zoodles 73

     5. Shrimp Stir-Fry with Vegetables 74

     6. Chickpea and Spinach Curry 75

Chapter 9 77

   Special Diets and Considerations 77

   RECIPES 77

     1. Quinoa and Black Bean Stuffed Bell Peppers (Gluten-Free, Vegetarian) 77

     2. Cauliflower Fried Rice (Low-Carb, Dairy-Free) 79

     3. Lemon Herb Baked Salmon (Paleo, Dairy-Free) 80

     4. Chickpea and Spinach Curry (Vegan, Gluten-Free) 81

5. Grilled Chicken with Avocado Salsa (Keto, Dairy-Free) 82

  6. Zucchini Noodles with Pesto and Cherry Tomatoes (Vegetarian, Gluten-Free) 83

Chapter 10 85

  Maintaining Your Weight Loss Journey 85

  Key Strategies for Maintaining Weight Loss 85

  Recipes 86

    1. Grilled Chicken and Quinoa Salad 86

    2. Baked Salmon with Asparagus 87

    3. Turkey and Vegetable Stir-Fry 88

    4. Lentil and Spinach Soup 89

    5. Shrimp and Avocado Lettuce Wraps 90

    6. Zucchini Noodles with Pesto 91

  Conclusion 93

    Key Takeaways 93

    Final Thoughts 94

INTRODUCTION

Welcome to *The Effective Weight Loss Cookbook*, your comprehensive guide to shedding pounds while savoring every bite. In a world where quick fixes and fad diets abound, this cookbook offers a sustainable, enjoyable approach to weight loss, focusing on real food and balanced nutrition.

Whether you're just starting your weight loss journey or looking to break through a plateau, this book is packed with recipes that are not only delicious but also tailored to help you reach your goals. We've combined the latest nutritional science with practical cooking techniques to create meals that are low in calories but high in flavor and satisfaction.

Each recipe in this cookbook is designed to support your weight loss efforts by using wholesome ingredients, balanced macronutrients, and mindful portion sizes. From energizing breakfasts and satisfying lunches to hearty dinners and guilt-free desserts, you'll find a variety of dishes that make healthy eating an exciting and achievable endeavor.

But this book is more than just a collection of recipes. It's a resource for building lasting habits that promote a healthier lifestyle. Alongside each recipe, you'll find tips on meal prepping, mindful eating, and understanding the nutritional value of your food. Our goal is to empower you with the knowledge and confidence to make informed choices that support your weight loss journey.

We believe that effective weight loss doesn't have to mean deprivation or monotony. With *The Effective Weight Loss Cookbook*, you'll discover that healthy eating can be a joyful and rewarding experience. So, grab your apron, stock your pantry, and get ready to embark on a culinary adventure that will transform the way you look at weight loss. Here's to delicious meals, a healthier you, and a journey well worth taking!

CHAPTER 1
INTRODUCTION TO EFFECTIVE WEIGHT LOSS

Understanding Effective Weight Loss

Weight loss is a multifaceted journey that requires a combination of a balanced diet, regular physical activity, and a positive mindset. The primary goal is not just to lose weight quickly, but to develop sustainable habits that promote long-term health and well-being. This chapter will guide you through the principles of effective weight loss, the importance of nutrition, and how to make the most out of this cookbook.

The Role of Nutrition in Weight Loss

Proper nutrition is the cornerstone of any successful weight loss plan. It involves consuming the right balance of macronutrients—proteins, fats, and carbohydrates—while also ensuring adequate intake of vitamins and minerals. This cookbook focuses on nutrient-dense recipes that are not only low in calories but also satisfying and delicious. By making informed food choices, you can manage your calorie intake without feeling deprived.

Importance of Meal Planning and Preparation

One of the most effective strategies for weight loss is meal planning and preparation. By planning your meals in advance, you can control portion sizes, avoid unhealthy food choices, and save time. This cookbook provides a variety of recipes that are easy to prepare and perfect for meal prepping. Each recipe includes detailed nutritional information to help you stay on track with your weight loss goals.

Staying Motivated and Consistent

Consistency is key when it comes to weight loss. It's important to set realistic goals, track your progress, and celebrate your achievements along the way. Staying motivated can be challenging, but remember that small, gradual changes often lead to the most significant results. Use this cookbook as a tool to support your weight loss journey and to find joy in cooking and eating healthy meals.

RECIPES

1. GRILLED CHICKEN WITH QUINOA AND VEGGIES

Ingredients:

- 2 boneless, skinless chicken breasts
- 1 cup quinoa
- 2 cups low-sodium chicken broth
- 1 red bell pepper, chopped
- 1 zucchini, sliced
- 1 tablespoon olive oil
- 1 teaspoon garlic powder
- Salt and pepper to taste

Prep Time: 15 minutes
Cooking Time: 30 minutes
Servings: 2

Instructions:

1. Preheat the grill to medium-high heat.
2. Season the chicken breasts with olive oil, garlic powder, salt, and pepper.
3. Grill the chicken for 6-7 minutes per side or until fully cooked.

4. In a saucepan, bring the chicken broth to a boil and add the quinoa. Reduce heat, cover, and simmer for 15 minutes.
5. In a skillet, sauté the red bell pepper and zucchini until tender.
6. Serve the grilled chicken over the quinoa and veggies.

2. BAKED SALMON WITH ASPARAGUS

Ingredients:

- 2 salmon fillets
- 1 bunch asparagus, trimmed
- 2 tablespoons olive oil
- 1 lemon, sliced
- 1 teaspoon dried dill
- Salt and pepper to taste

Prep Time: 10 minutes
Cooking Time: 20 minutes
Servings: 2

Instructions:

1. Preheat the oven to 400°F (200°C).
2. Place the salmon fillets and asparagus on a baking sheet.

3. Drizzle with olive oil and season with dill, salt, and pepper.
4. Arrange lemon slices on top of the salmon.
5. Bake for 20 minutes or until the salmon is cooked through and the asparagus is tender.

3. TURKEY AND VEGETABLE STIR-FRY

Ingredients:

- 1 pound ground turkey
- 1 red bell pepper, sliced
- 1 yellow bell pepper, sliced
- 1 cup broccoli florets
- 1 carrot, julienned
- 2 tablespoons soy sauce (low sodium)
- 1 tablespoon sesame oil
- 2 cloves garlic, minced
- 1 teaspoon ginger, minced

Prep Time: 15 minutes
Cooking Time: 15 minutes
Servings: 4

Instructions:

1. In a large skillet or wok, heat sesame oil over medium-high heat.

2. Add garlic and ginger, and sauté for 1 minute.
3. Add the ground turkey and cook until browned.
4. Add the bell peppers, broccoli, and carrot. Stir-fry for 5-7 minutes.
5. Pour in the soy sauce and cook for another 2-3 minutes.
6. Serve hot.

4. VEGGIE-PACKED CAULIFLOWER RICE BOWL

Ingredients:

- 1 medium head of cauliflower, grated into rice-sized pieces
- 1 cup cherry tomatoes, halved
- 1 cucumber, diced
- 1 avocado, sliced
- 1/4 cup red onion, finely chopped
- 2 tablespoons olive oil
- 1 tablespoon lemon juice
- Salt and pepper to taste

Prep Time: 15 minutes
Cooking Time: 10 minutes
Servings: 2

Instructions:

1. Heat olive oil in a large skillet over medium heat.
2. Add the grated cauliflower and cook for 5-7 minutes until tender.
3. In a bowl, combine the cooked cauliflower rice with cherry tomatoes, cucumber, avocado, and red onion.
4. Drizzle with lemon juice and season with salt and pepper.
5. Serve immediately.

5. SPAGHETTI SQUASH WITH TOMATO BASIL SAUCE

Ingredients:

- 1 medium spaghetti squash
- 2 cups cherry tomatoes, halved
- 2 cloves garlic, minced
- 2 tablespoons olive oil
- 1/4 cup fresh basil, chopped
- Salt and pepper to taste

Prep Time: 10 minutes
Cooking Time: 40 minutes
Servings: 4

Instructions:

1. Preheat the oven to 375°F (190°C).
2. Cut the spaghetti squash in half lengthwise and remove the seeds.
3. Drizzle with olive oil, season with salt and pepper, and place cut side down on a baking sheet.
4. Bake for 40 minutes or until the squash is tender.
5. In a skillet, heat olive oil and sauté garlic until fragrant.
6. Add cherry tomatoes and cook until they begin to break down.
7. Scrape the spaghetti squash into strands and add to the skillet.
8. Toss with fresh basil and serve hot.

6. CHICKEN AND AVOCADO SALAD

Ingredients:

- 2 cups cooked, shredded chicken breast
- 1 avocado, diced
- 1 cup cherry tomatoes, halved
- 1/2 red onion, thinly sliced
- 2 cups mixed greens
- 2 tablespoons olive oil
- 1 tablespoon balsamic vinegar
- Salt and pepper to taste

Prep Time: 15 minutes
Cooking Time: 0 minutes
Servings: 2

Instructions:

1. In a large bowl, combine the shredded chicken, avocado, cherry tomatoes, red onion, and mixed greens.
2. In a small bowl, whisk together olive oil, balsamic vinegar, salt, and pepper.
3. Pour the dressing over the salad and toss to combine.
4. Serve immediately.

CHAPTER 2

ENERGIZING BREAKFASTS

RECIPES

1. AVOCADO TOAST WITH POACHED EGG

Ingredients:

- 1 ripe avocado
- 2 slices whole grain bread
- 2 large eggs
- 1 tbsp lemon juice
- Salt and pepper to taste
- Red pepper flakes (optional)
- Fresh parsley, chopped (optional)

Prep Time: 10 minutes
Cooking Time: 5 minutes
Servings: 2

Instructions:

1. Toast the whole grain bread slices until golden brown.
2. While the bread is toasting, bring a pot of water to a gentle simmer.
3. Crack the eggs into separate small bowls.
4. Create a gentle whirlpool in the water and carefully slide the eggs into the water.
5. Poach the eggs for 3-4 minutes until the whites are set but the yolks are still runny.
6. While the eggs are poaching, mash the avocado in a bowl and mix with lemon juice, salt, and pepper.
7. Spread the avocado mixture evenly on the toasted bread.
8. Top each toast with a poached egg.
9. Sprinkle with red pepper flakes and chopped parsley if desired.
10. Serve immediately.

2. GREEK YOGURT PARFAIT

Ingredients:

- 2 cups Greek yogurt
- 1 cup mixed berries (strawberries, blueberries, raspberries)

- 1/4 cup granola
- 2 tbsp honey
- 1 tbsp chia seeds
- Fresh mint leaves (optional)

Prep Time: 10 minutes
Cooking Time: 0 minutes
Servings: 2

Instructions:

1. In two glasses or bowls, add a layer of Greek yogurt at the bottom.
2. Top the yogurt with a layer of mixed berries.
3. Add a sprinkle of granola over the berries.
4. Repeat the layers until all ingredients are used up.
5. Drizzle honey over the top layer.
6. Sprinkle with chia seeds.
7. Garnish with fresh mint leaves if desired.
8. Serve immediately or refrigerate until ready to eat.

3. SPINACH AND FETA OMELETTE

Ingredients:

- 4 large eggs
- 1 cup fresh spinach, chopped
- 1/4 cup feta cheese, crumbled
- 1/4 cup onion, finely chopped
- 1 tbsp olive oil

- Salt and pepper to taste

Prep Time: 5 minutes
Cooking Time: 10 minutes
Servings: 2

Instructions:

1. In a bowl, whisk the eggs with a pinch of salt and pepper.
2. Heat olive oil in a non-stick skillet over medium heat.
3. Add the chopped onion and sauté until translucent.
4. Add the spinach and cook until wilted.
5. Pour the beaten eggs into the skillet and let them cook undisturbed for a minute.
6. Sprinkle the feta cheese over the eggs.
7. Cook until the eggs are set but still slightly runny on top.
8. Fold the omelette in half and cook for another minute.
9. Serve hot with a side of fresh tomatoes or toast.

4. BERRY AND BANANA SMOOTHIE BOWL

Ingredients:

- 1 banana, sliced and frozen
- 1 cup mixed berries (blueberries, strawberries, raspberries)

- 1/2 cup unsweetened almond milk
- 1 tbsp almond butter
- 1 tbsp chia seeds
- 1/4 cup granola
- Fresh berries and banana slices for topping

Prep Time: 5 minutes
Cooking Time: 5 minutes
Servings: 2

Instructions:

1. In a blender, combine the frozen banana, mixed berries, almond milk, almond butter, and chia seeds.
2. Blend until smooth and creamy.
3. Pour the smoothie mixture into two bowls.
4. Top with fresh berries, banana slices, and granola.
5. Serve immediately with a spoon.

5. QUINOA BREAKFAST BOWL

Ingredients:

- 1/2 cup quinoa
- 1 cup water
- 1/2 cup almond milk
- 1 tbsp maple syrup
- 1/2 tsp cinnamon
- 1/4 cup chopped nuts (almonds, walnuts)
- 1/4 cup dried fruit (raisins, cranberries)

- Fresh berries for topping

Prep Time: 5 minutes
Cooking Time: 15 minutes
Servings: 2

Instructions:

1. Rinse the quinoa under cold water.
2. In a medium saucepan, combine the quinoa and water. Bring to a boil.
3. Reduce heat to low, cover, and simmer for 10-12 minutes until the quinoa is cooked and water is absorbed.
4. Stir in the almond milk, maple syrup, and cinnamon.
5. Cook for another 2-3 minutes until heated through.
6. Divide the quinoa mixture between two bowls.
7. Top with chopped nuts, dried fruit, and fresh berries.
8. Serve warm.

6. VEGGIE-PACKED BREAKFAST BURRITO

Ingredients:

- 4 large eggs
- 1/4 cup milk
- 1 tbsp olive oil
- 1/2 cup bell peppers, diced

- 1/2 cup zucchini, diced
- 1/4 cup onion, finely chopped
- 1/4 cup cheddar cheese, shredded
- 2 whole wheat tortillas
- Salt and pepper to taste
- Salsa and avocado slices for serving (optional)

Prep Time: 10 minutes
Cooking Time: 10 minutes
Servings: 2

Instructions:

1. In a bowl, whisk the eggs with milk, salt, and pepper.
2. Heat olive oil in a large skillet over medium heat.
3. Add the diced bell peppers, zucchini, and onion. Sauté until tender.
4. Pour the egg mixture into the skillet and cook, stirring frequently, until the eggs are scrambled and fully cooked.
5. Sprinkle the shredded cheddar cheese over the eggs and stir until melted.
6. Warm the whole wheat tortillas in a separate skillet or microwave.
7. Divide the egg mixture between the two tortillas.
8. Roll up the tortillas to form burritos.
9. Serve with salsa and avocado slices if desired.

CHAPTER 3

SATISFYING LUNCHES

Lunchtime is a pivotal moment in your day, especially when you're focusing on weight loss. It's important to choose meals that are not only delicious and satisfying but also nutritionally balanced to keep you full and energized throughout the afternoon. The following recipes are crafted to help you achieve your weight loss goals while enjoying every bite. Each dish is designed to be low in calories, high in nutrients, and easy to prepare.

RECIPES

1. QUINOA AND BLACK BEAN SALAD

Ingredients:

- 1 cup quinoa, rinsed
- 2 cups water
- 1 can (15 oz) black beans, drained and rinsed
- 1 cup cherry tomatoes, halved

- 1 avocado, diced
- 1 red bell pepper, diced
- 1/4 cup red onion, finely chopped
- 1/4 cup fresh cilantro, chopped
- 1/4 cup fresh lime juice
- 2 tbsp olive oil
- 1 tsp cumin
- Salt and pepper to taste

Prep Time: 15 minutes
Cooking Time: 15 minutes
Servings: 4

Instructions:

1. In a medium pot, bring quinoa and water to a boil. Reduce heat, cover, and simmer for 15 minutes or until quinoa is tender and water is absorbed.
2. In a large bowl, combine cooked quinoa, black beans, cherry tomatoes, avocado, red bell pepper, red onion, and cilantro.
3. In a small bowl, whisk together lime juice, olive oil, cumin, salt, and pepper. Pour over the quinoa mixture and toss to coat.
4. Serve immediately or refrigerate for up to 2 days.

2. TURKEY AND AVOCADO LETTUCE WRAPS

Ingredients:

- 12 large lettuce leaves (romaine or iceberg)
- 1 lb ground turkey
- 1 tbsp olive oil
- 1 red bell pepper, diced
- 1 small red onion, diced
- 2 cloves garlic, minced
- 1 tsp chili powder
- 1 tsp cumin
- 1/2 tsp paprika
- Salt and pepper to taste
- 1 avocado, sliced
- 1/4 cup fresh cilantro, chopped

Prep Time: 10 minutes
Cooking Time: 15 minutes
Servings: 4

Instructions:

1. Heat olive oil in a large skillet over medium heat. Add garlic, red onion, and red bell pepper, and cook until softened, about 5 minutes.
2. Add ground turkey and cook until browned, breaking it up with a spoon, about 7-10 minutes.
3. Stir in chili powder, cumin, paprika, salt, and pepper. Cook for another 2 minutes.
4. Remove from heat and let cool slightly. Spoon turkey mixture into lettuce leaves.
5. Top with avocado slices and cilantro. Serve immediately.

3. GRILLED CHICKEN AND VEGGIE SKEWERS

Ingredients:

- 2 boneless, skinless chicken breasts, cut into 1-inch cubes
- 1 zucchini, sliced
- 1 red bell pepper, cut into squares
- 1 yellow bell pepper, cut into squares
- 1 red onion, cut into wedges
- 1/4 cup olive oil
- 2 tbsp fresh lemon juice
- 2 cloves garlic, minced
- 1 tsp dried oregano
- Salt and pepper to taste
- Wooden skewers, soaked in water for 30 minutes

Prep Time: 20 minutes
Cooking Time: 15 minutes
Servings: 4

Instructions:

1. In a large bowl, combine olive oil, lemon juice, garlic, oregano, salt, and pepper.
2. Add chicken and vegetables to the bowl, tossing to coat. Marinate for at least 15 minutes.
3. Preheat grill to medium-high heat. Thread chicken and vegetables onto skewers.

4. Grill skewers for 10-15 minutes, turning occasionally, until chicken is cooked through and vegetables are tender.
5. Serve immediately.

4. CAULIFLOWER FRIED RICE

Ingredients:

- 1 medium head cauliflower, cut into florets
- 1 tbsp olive oil
- 1 cup frozen peas and carrots, thawed
- 1 small onion, diced
- 2 cloves garlic, minced
- 2 large eggs, beaten
- 3 tbsp low-sodium soy sauce
- 1 tbsp sesame oil
- 2 green onions, sliced
- Salt and pepper to taste

Prep Time: 10 minutes
Cooking Time: 15 minutes
Servings: 4

Instructions:

1. In a food processor, pulse cauliflower florets until they resemble rice grains.
2. Heat olive oil in a large skillet over medium heat. Add onion and garlic, and cook until fragrant, about 2 minutes.

3. Add peas and carrots, and cook for another 2-3 minutes.
4. Push vegetables to one side of the skillet and pour beaten eggs into the other side. Scramble the eggs until cooked through.
5. Add cauliflower rice to the skillet, mixing with vegetables and eggs. Cook for 5-7 minutes, until cauliflower is tender.
6. Stir in soy sauce, sesame oil, salt, and pepper. Top with green onions and serve.

5. LENTIL AND SPINACH SOUP

Ingredients:

- 1 cup green lentils, rinsed
- 1 tbsp olive oil
- 1 large onion, diced
- 2 carrots, diced
- 2 celery stalks, diced
- 2 cloves garlic, minced
- 1 tsp cumin
- 1/2 tsp turmeric
- 8 cups vegetable broth
- 4 cups fresh spinach
- Salt and pepper to taste

Prep Time: 10 minutes
Cooking Time: 30 minutes
Servings: 4

Instructions:

1. In a large pot, heat olive oil over medium heat. Add onion, carrots, and celery, and cook until softened, about 5 minutes.
2. Add garlic, cumin, and turmeric, and cook for another minute.
3. Add lentils and vegetable broth. Bring to a boil, then reduce heat and simmer for 20-25 minutes, until lentils are tender.
4. Stir in spinach and cook until wilted, about 2 minutes. Season with salt and pepper.
5. Serve hot.

6. GREEK YOGURT CHICKEN SALAD

Ingredients:

- 2 cups cooked chicken breast, shredded
- 1 cup plain Greek yogurt
- 1/2 cup celery, diced
- 1/2 cup red grapes, halved
- 1/4 cup red onion, finely chopped
- 1/4 cup fresh parsley, chopped
- 1 tbsp fresh lemon juice
- 1 tsp Dijon mustard
- Salt and pepper to taste
- Lettuce leaves for serving

Prep Time: 15 minutes
Cooking Time: 0 minutes
Servings: 4

Instructions:

1. In a large bowl, combine Greek yogurt, lemon juice, Dijon mustard, salt, and pepper.
2. Add shredded chicken, celery, grapes, red onion, and parsley. Mix until well combined.
3. Serve chicken salad in lettuce leaves or on whole-grain bread.
4. Enjoy immediately or refrigerate for up to 2 days.

CHAPTER 4

DELICIOUS DINNERS

In this chapter, we will explore a variety of delicious and nutritious dinner recipes designed to help you on your weight loss journey. Each recipe is crafted to be both satisfying and healthful, ensuring you can enjoy flavorful meals without compromising your goals. These dinners are easy to prepare and perfect for any night of the week.

RECIPES

1. LEMON HERB GRILLED CHICKEN

Ingredients:

- 4 boneless, skinless chicken breasts
- 2 tablespoons olive oil
- 3 tablespoons lemon juice
- 1 tablespoon chopped fresh rosemary
- 1 tablespoon chopped fresh thyme
- 2 garlic cloves, minced

- Salt and pepper to taste

Prep Time: 10 minutes
Cooking Time: 15 minutes
Servings: 4

Instructions:

1. In a small bowl, combine olive oil, lemon juice, rosemary, thyme, garlic, salt, and pepper.
2. Place the chicken breasts in a resealable plastic bag and pour the marinade over them. Seal the bag and refrigerate for at least 30 minutes.
3. Preheat the grill to medium-high heat.
4. Remove the chicken from the marinade and discard the marinade.
5. Grill the chicken for 6-7 minutes on each side, or until the internal temperature reaches 165°F (75°C).
6. Serve the grilled chicken with a side of steamed vegetables or a fresh salad.

2. QUINOA STUFFED BELL PEPPERS

Ingredients:

- 4 large bell peppers (any color), tops cut off and seeds removed
- 1 cup cooked quinoa
- 1 can (15 oz) black beans, rinsed and drained

- 1 cup corn kernels (fresh or frozen)
- 1 cup diced tomatoes
- 1/2 cup diced onion
- 1 teaspoon cumin
- 1 teaspoon chili powder
- Salt and pepper to taste
- 1/2 cup shredded low-fat cheddar cheese (optional)
- Fresh cilantro for garnish

Prep Time: 15 minutes
Cooking Time: 30 minutes
Servings: 4

Instructions:

1. Preheat the oven to 375°F (190°C).
2. In a large bowl, combine cooked quinoa, black beans, corn, tomatoes, onion, cumin, chili powder, salt, and pepper.
3. Stuff each bell pepper with the quinoa mixture and place them in a baking dish.
4. Cover the dish with foil and bake for 25 minutes.
5. If using, remove the foil and sprinkle shredded cheese on top of each pepper. Bake for an additional 5 minutes, until the cheese is melted.
6. Garnish with fresh cilantro before serving.

3. BAKED SALMON WITH ASPARAGUS

Ingredients:

- 4 salmon fillets (about 6 oz each)
- 1 pound asparagus, trimmed
- 2 tablespoons olive oil
- 2 tablespoons lemon juice
- 1 tablespoon chopped fresh dill
- Salt and pepper to taste
- Lemon wedges for serving

Prep Time: 10 minutes
Cooking Time: 20 minutes
Servings: 4

Instructions:

1. Preheat the oven to 400°F (200°C).
2. Place the salmon fillets and asparagus on a baking sheet lined with parchment paper.
3. Drizzle olive oil and lemon juice over the salmon and asparagus. Season with dill, salt, and pepper.
4. Bake for 15-20 minutes, until the salmon is cooked through and flakes easily with a fork.
5. Serve the salmon and asparagus with lemon wedges.

4. SPAGHETTI SQUASH WITH TURKEY MARINARA

Ingredients:

- 1 large spaghetti squash
- 1 tablespoon olive oil
- 1 pound ground turkey
- 1 onion, diced
- 2 garlic cloves, minced
- 1 can (28 oz) crushed tomatoes
- 1 teaspoon dried oregano
- 1 teaspoon dried basil
- Salt and pepper to taste
- Fresh basil for garnish

Prep Time: 15 minutes
Cooking Time: 45 minutes
Servings: 4

Instructions:

1. Preheat the oven to 375°F (190°C).
2. Cut the spaghetti squash in half lengthwise and scoop out the seeds.
3. Drizzle the cut sides of the squash with olive oil and season with salt and pepper. Place cut side down on a baking sheet and bake for 40-45 minutes, until tender.
4. While the squash is baking, heat a large skillet over medium heat and cook the ground turkey until browned.
5. Add the onion and garlic to the skillet and cook until softened.
6. Stir in the crushed tomatoes, oregano, basil, salt, and pepper. Simmer for 15 minutes.

7. When the squash is done, use a fork to scrape out the strands into a bowl.
8. Serve the spaghetti squash topped with turkey marinara sauce and garnish with fresh basil.

5. CAULIFLOWER FRIED RICE

Ingredients:

- 1 medium head cauliflower, riced
- 1 tablespoon sesame oil
- 2 eggs, lightly beaten
- 1 cup frozen peas and carrots
- 1/2 cup diced onion
- 2 garlic cloves, minced
- 3 tablespoons low-sodium soy sauce
- 2 green onions, chopped

Prep Time: 10 minutes
Cooking Time: 15 minutes
Servings: 4

Instructions:

1. Heat a large skillet or wok over medium-high heat and add sesame oil.

2. Add the beaten eggs and scramble until fully cooked. Remove from the skillet and set aside.
3. In the same skillet, add the diced onion and garlic, and sauté until fragrant.
4. Add the frozen peas and carrots and cook until tender.
5. Stir in the riced cauliflower and soy sauce. Cook for 5-7 minutes, until the cauliflower is tender.
6. Return the scrambled eggs to the skillet and stir to combine.
7. Garnish with chopped green onions before serving.

6. ZUCCHINI NOODLES WITH PESTO AND GRILLED SHRIMP

Ingredients:

- 4 medium zucchinis, spiralized
- 1 pound large shrimp, peeled and deveined
- 2 tablespoons olive oil, divided
- 1/4 cup basil pesto
- 1/4 cup grated Parmesan cheese
- Salt and pepper to taste
- Cherry tomatoes for garnish (optional)

Prep Time: 15 minutes
Cooking Time: 10 minutes
Servings: 4

Instructions:

1. Heat 1 tablespoon of olive oil in a large skillet over medium-high heat.
2. Add the shrimp and cook for 2-3 minutes on each side, until pink and opaque. Remove from the skillet and set aside.
3. In the same skillet, add the remaining olive oil and zucchini noodles. Cook for 2-3 minutes, until slightly tender.
4. Remove the skillet from the heat and toss the zucchini noodles with basil pesto.
5. Divide the zucchini noodles among four plates and top with grilled shrimp.
6. Sprinkle with grated Parmesan cheese and garnish with cherry tomatoes if desired.

CHAPTER 5

SMART SNACKS AND APPETIZERS

In "The Effective Weight Loss Cookbook," we recognize the importance of smart snacking and appetizing starters to maintain your weight loss journey while satisfying your cravings. These snacks and appetizers are designed to be nutritious, low-calorie, and delicious, ensuring you can enjoy without guilt. Here are six carefully curated recipes to add to your healthy eating repertoire.

RECIPES

1. CUCUMBER HUMMUS BITES

Ingredients:

- 1 large cucumber
- 1 cup hummus
- 1/4 cup cherry tomatoes, diced
- 1/4 cup feta cheese, crumbled

- 1 tbsp fresh dill, chopped

Prep Time: 15 minutes
Servings: 4

Instructions:

1. Slice the cucumber into 1/2-inch thick rounds.
2. Scoop a small amount of seeds out of each cucumber slice to create a small cavity.
3. Fill each cucumber slice with hummus.
4. Top with diced cherry tomatoes, feta cheese, and a sprinkle of fresh dill.
5. Serve immediately or refrigerate until ready to serve.

2. GREEK YOGURT AND BERRY PARFAIT

Ingredients:

- 1 cup Greek yogurt
- 1/2 cup mixed berries (blueberries, strawberries, raspberries)
- 1 tbsp honey
- 1 tbsp chia seeds
- 1/4 cup granola (optional for added crunch)

Prep Time: 10 minutes
Servings: 2

Instructions:

1. Layer half of the Greek yogurt in the bottom of two serving glasses.
2. Add a layer of mixed berries.
3. Drizzle with honey and sprinkle with chia seeds.
4. Repeat the layers with the remaining yogurt, berries, honey, and chia seeds.
5. Top with granola if desired. Serve immediately.

3. AVOCADO AND BLACK BEAN SALSA

Ingredients:

- 1 ripe avocado, diced
- 1 can (15 oz) black beans, rinsed and drained
- 1/2 cup corn kernels (fresh or frozen)
- 1/2 cup cherry tomatoes, halved
- 1/4 cup red onion, finely chopped
- 1/4 cup cilantro, chopped
- Juice of 1 lime
- Salt and pepper to taste

Prep Time: 15 minutes
Servings: 4

Instructions:

1. In a large bowl, combine the diced avocado, black beans, corn, cherry tomatoes, red onion, and cilantro.
2. Squeeze the lime juice over the mixture and gently toss to combine.
3. Season with salt and pepper to taste.
4. Serve with whole-grain tortilla chips or as a topping for salads or grilled chicken.

4. BAKED ZUCCHINI CHIPS

Ingredients:

- 2 medium zucchinis, thinly sliced
- 1 tbsp olive oil
- 1/4 cup grated Parmesan cheese
- 1/2 tsp garlic powder
- 1/2 tsp paprika
- Salt and pepper to taste

Prep Time: 10 minutes
Cooking Time: 25 minutes
Servings: 4

Instructions:

1. Preheat the oven to 400°F (200°C) and line a baking sheet with parchment paper.

2. In a large bowl, toss the zucchini slices with olive oil.
3. In a small bowl, combine the Parmesan cheese, garlic powder, paprika, salt, and pepper.
4. Sprinkle the cheese mixture over the zucchini slices and toss to coat evenly.
5. Arrange the zucchini slices in a single layer on the prepared baking sheet.
6. Bake for 20-25 minutes, or until golden and crispy.
7. Allow to cool slightly before serving.

5. SPICY ROASTED CHICKPEAS

Ingredients:

- 1 can (15 oz) chickpeas, rinsed and drained
- 1 tbsp olive oil
- 1 tsp smoked paprika
- 1/2 tsp cayenne pepper
- 1/2 tsp garlic powder
- Salt to taste

Prep Time: 5 minutes
Cooking Time: 35 minutes
Servings: 4

Instructions:

1. Preheat the oven to 400°F (200°C) and line a baking sheet with parchment paper.

2. Pat the chickpeas dry with a paper towel.
3. In a bowl, toss the chickpeas with olive oil, smoked paprika, cayenne pepper, garlic powder, and salt.
4. Spread the chickpeas in a single layer on the prepared baking sheet.
5. Roast for 30-35 minutes, shaking the pan halfway through, until the chickpeas are crispy.
6. Allow to cool slightly before serving.

6. STUFFED MINI BELL PEPPERS

Ingredients:

- 12 mini bell peppers
- 1 cup quinoa, cooked and cooled
- 1/2 cup black beans, rinsed and drained
- 1/2 cup corn kernels (fresh or frozen)
- 1/4 cup red onion, finely chopped
- 1/4 cup cilantro, chopped
- 1/2 cup salsa
- 1/4 cup shredded cheese (optional)
- Salt and pepper to taste

Prep Time: 15 minutes
Cooking Time: 10 minutes
Servings: 6

Instructions:

1. Preheat the oven to 375°F (190°C).

2. Slice the tops off the mini bell peppers and remove the seeds.
3. In a large bowl, combine the cooked quinoa, black beans, corn, red onion, cilantro, and salsa.
4. Season with salt and pepper to taste.
5. Stuff each mini bell pepper with the quinoa mixture.
6. Place the stuffed peppers on a baking sheet and sprinkle with shredded cheese if desired.
7. Bake for 10 minutes, or until the peppers are tender and the cheese is melted.
8. Serve warm or at room temperature.

CHAPTER 6

GUILT-FREE DESSERTS

In this chapter, you'll find a collection of delightful desserts that are both delicious and healthy. These recipes are designed to satisfy your sweet tooth without derailing your weight loss goals. Enjoy these guilt-free treats that are low in calories, sugar, and unhealthy fats.

RECIPES

1. CHOCOLATE AVOCADO MOUSSE

Ingredients:

- 2 ripe avocados
- 1/4 cup unsweetened cocoa powder
- 1/4 cup honey or maple syrup
- 1/4 cup almond milk
- 1 tsp vanilla extract
- A pinch of sea salt

Prep Time: 10 minutes
Cooking Time: None
Servings: 4

Instructions:

1. Cut the avocados in half, remove the pits, and scoop out the flesh.
2. In a blender, combine the avocado, cocoa powder, honey or maple syrup, almond milk, vanilla extract, and sea salt.
3. Blend until smooth and creamy.
4. Divide the mousse into four serving dishes.
5. Chill in the refrigerator for at least 30 minutes before serving.

2. GREEK YOGURT BERRY PARFAIT

Ingredients:

- 2 cups non-fat Greek yogurt
- 1 cup mixed berries (strawberries, blueberries, raspberries)
- 1/4 cup granola (optional)
- 2 tbsp honey
- 1 tsp vanilla extract

Prep Time: 10 minutes
Cooking Time: None
Servings: 2

Instructions:

1. In a bowl, mix the Greek yogurt with honey and vanilla extract.
2. In two serving glasses, layer half of the yogurt mixture, followed by half of the berries.
3. Repeat the layers with the remaining yogurt and berries.
4. Top each parfait with a sprinkle of granola if desired.
5. Serve immediately or refrigerate until ready to eat.

3. BAKED APPLES WITH CINNAMON

Ingredients:

- 4 large apples
- 1/4 cup chopped nuts (walnuts or pecans)
- 1/4 cup raisins
- 1 tsp ground cinnamon
- 2 tbsp honey
- 1/4 cup water

Prep Time: 10 minutes
Cooking Time: 30 minutes
Servings: 4

Instructions:

1. Preheat the oven to 375°F (190°C).

2. Core the apples, leaving the bottom intact to create a well.
3. In a small bowl, mix the nuts, raisins, and cinnamon.
4. Stuff the mixture into the apples and place them in a baking dish.
5. Drizzle honey over the apples and pour water into the bottom of the dish.
6. Bake for 30 minutes or until the apples are tender.
7. Serve warm.

4. CHIA SEED PUDDING

Ingredients:

- 1/4 cup chia seeds
- 1 cup almond milk
- 1 tbsp honey or maple syrup
- 1/2 tsp vanilla extract
- Fresh fruit for topping (optional)

Prep Time: 5 minutes
Cooking Time: None (chill for 2 hours or overnight)
Servings: 2

Instructions:

1. In a bowl, mix chia seeds, almond milk, honey or maple syrup, and vanilla extract.
2. Stir well to combine.

3. Cover and refrigerate for at least 2 hours or overnight until the mixture thickens.
4. Stir again before serving.
5. Top with fresh fruit if desired.

5. BANANA OAT COOKIES

Ingredients:

- 2 ripe bananas
- 1 cup rolled oats
- 1/4 cup dark chocolate chips
- 1/4 cup chopped nuts (optional)
- 1 tsp vanilla extract

Prep Time: 10 minutes
Cooking Time: 15 minutes
Servings: 12 cookies

Instructions:

1. Preheat the oven to 350°F (175°C).
2. In a bowl, mash the bananas until smooth.
3. Stir in the oats, dark chocolate chips, nuts (if using), and vanilla extract.
4. Drop spoonfuls of the mixture onto a baking sheet lined with parchment paper.
5. Bake for 12-15 minutes or until golden brown.
6. Allow to cool on a wire rack before serving.

6. LEMON YOGURT CAKE

Ingredients:

- 1 cup whole wheat flour
- 1/2 cup almond flour
- 1/2 tsp baking soda
- 1/2 tsp baking powder
- 1/4 tsp salt
- 2 eggs
- 1/2 cup honey
- 1 cup plain Greek yogurt
- 1/4 cup fresh lemon juice
- Zest of 1 lemon
- 1 tsp vanilla extract

Prep Time: 15 minutes
Cooking Time: 30 minutes
Servings: 8

Instructions:

1. Preheat the oven to 350°F (175°C). Grease a 9-inch round cake pan.
2. In a bowl, whisk together the whole wheat flour, almond flour, baking soda, baking powder, and salt.
3. In another bowl, beat the eggs and honey until well combined.
4. Stir in the Greek yogurt, lemon juice, lemon zest, and vanilla extract.

5. Gradually add the dry ingredients to the wet ingredients, mixing until just combined.
6. Pour the batter into the prepared cake pan.
7. Bake for 25-30 minutes or until a toothpick inserted into the center comes out clean.
8. Allow the cake to cool in the pan for 10 minutes before transferring to a wire rack to cool completely.

CHAPTER 7

SMOOTHIES AND BEVERAGES

Smoothies and beverages can be a delightful and nutritious way to support your weight loss journey. Whether you're starting your day with a nutrient-packed smoothie, enjoying a refreshing drink during the afternoon, or winding down with a calming beverage, these recipes will help you stay on track while satisfying your taste buds.

RECIPES

1. GREEN DETOX SMOOTHIE

Ingredients:

- 1 cup spinach leaves
- 1 cup kale leaves
- 1 green apple, cored and chopped
- 1 banana

- 1/2 cucumber, chopped
- 1 tablespoon chia seeds
- 1 cup coconut water
- 1 tablespoon lemon juice

Prep Time: 10 minutes
Cooking Time: None
Servings: 2

Instructions:

1. Place all ingredients in a blender.
2. Blend until smooth and creamy.
3. Pour into glasses and serve immediately.

2. BERRY PROTEIN SMOOTHIE

Ingredients:

- 1 cup mixed berries (strawberries, blueberries, raspberries)
- 1 scoop vanilla protein powder
- 1 cup unsweetened almond milk
- 1/2 banana
- 1 tablespoon flax seeds
- 1/2 cup Greek yogurt

Prep Time: 10 minutes
Cooking Time: None
Servings: 2

Instructions:

1. Combine all ingredients in a blender.
2. Blend until smooth.
3. Pour into glasses and enjoy.

3. TROPICAL MANGO SMOOTHIE

Ingredients:

- 1 cup frozen mango chunks
- 1/2 cup pineapple chunks
- 1/2 cup coconut milk
- 1/2 cup orange juice
- 1 tablespoon honey
- 1/4 teaspoon turmeric powder

Prep Time: 10 minutes
Cooking Time: None
Servings: 2

Instructions:

1. Add all ingredients to a blender.
2. Blend until smooth.
3. Serve immediately.

4. MATCHA GREEN TEA LATTE

Ingredients:

- 1 teaspoon matcha green tea powder
- 1 cup unsweetened almond milk
- 1 tablespoon hot water
- 1 teaspoon honey (optional)

Prep Time: 5 minutes
Cooking Time: 5 minutes
Servings: 1

Instructions:

1. In a small bowl, whisk the matcha powder with hot water until smooth.
2. Heat almond milk in a saucepan until warm (do not boil).
3. Pour the matcha mixture into a mug, add warm almond milk, and stir well.
4. Sweeten with honey if desired.

5. CUCUMBER MINT DETOX WATER

Ingredients:

- 1 cucumber, thinly sliced
- 10-12 fresh mint leaves
- 1 lemon, thinly sliced
- 2 liters water

Prep Time: 5 minutes
Cooking Time: None
Servings: 8

Instructions:

1. In a large pitcher, combine cucumber slices, mint leaves, and lemon slices.
2. Fill the pitcher with water.
3. Let it sit in the refrigerator for at least 2 hours before serving.

6. GOLDEN MILK

Ingredients:

- 1 cup unsweetened almond milk
- 1/2 teaspoon turmeric powder
- 1/4 teaspoon ground ginger
- 1/4 teaspoon ground cinnamon
- 1 teaspoon honey or maple syrup
- A pinch of black pepper

Prep Time: 5 minutes
Cooking Time: 5 minutes
Servings: 1

Instructions:

1. In a small saucepan, combine almond milk, turmeric, ginger, cinnamon, and black pepper.
2. Heat over medium heat until warm, stirring frequently.
3. Remove from heat and stir in honey or maple syrup.
4. Pour into a mug and enjoy warm.

CHAPTER 8

MEAL PLANNING AND PREP

Effective meal planning and preparation are key strategies for successful weight loss. By planning your meals in advance, you can make healthier food choices, save time, and avoid the temptation of unhealthy snacks. This chapter provides tips on meal planning and prep, along with six main course recipes designed to support your weight loss journey.

TIPS FOR EFFECTIVE MEAL PLANNING AND PREP

1. **Plan Ahead**: Dedicate a specific day each week to plan your meals. Make a shopping list based on your meal plan to ensure you have all necessary ingredients.
2. **Batch Cooking**: Prepare large portions of meals that can be divided into servings and stored for later. This saves time and ensures you always have a healthy meal ready.

3. **Portion Control**: Use meal prep containers to portion out your meals. This helps control portion sizes and prevents overeating.
4. **Variety**: Include a variety of foods in your meal plan to ensure you're getting a balanced diet and to prevent boredom.
5. **Healthy Ingredients**: Focus on whole, nutrient-dense foods such as lean proteins, whole grains, vegetables, and fruits.

RECIPES

1. GRILLED LEMON HERB CHICKEN

Ingredients:

- 4 boneless, skinless chicken breasts
- 1/4 cup olive oil
- Juice of 2 lemons
- 3 cloves garlic, minced
- 1 tsp dried oregano
- 1 tsp dried thyme
- Salt and pepper to taste

Prep Time: 10 minutes
Cooking Time: 20 minutes
Servings: 4

Instructions:

1. In a bowl, mix olive oil, lemon juice, garlic, oregano, thyme, salt, and pepper.
2. Place chicken breasts in a resealable bag and pour the marinade over them. Marinate for at least 30 minutes.
3. Preheat grill to medium-high heat.
4. Grill chicken for 6-7 minutes on each side or until fully cooked.
5. Serve with a side of steamed vegetables or a salad.

2. QUINOA AND BLACK BEAN SALAD

Ingredients:

- 1 cup quinoa
- 2 cups water
- 1 can (15 oz) black beans, rinsed and drained
- 1 cup cherry tomatoes, halved
- 1 avocado, diced
- 1/4 cup red onion, finely chopped
- 1/4 cup cilantro, chopped
- 2 tbsp olive oil
- Juice of 1 lime
- Salt and pepper to taste

Prep Time: 15 minutes
Cooking Time: 15 minutes
Servings: 4

Instructions:

1. Rinse quinoa under cold water. In a pot, bring quinoa and water to a boil. Reduce heat, cover, and simmer for 15 minutes or until water is absorbed. Let cool.
2. In a large bowl, combine cooked quinoa, black beans, cherry tomatoes, avocado, red onion, and cilantro.
3. In a small bowl, whisk together olive oil, lime juice, salt, and pepper. Pour over the salad and toss to combine.
4. Serve immediately or refrigerate for later.

3. BAKED SALMON WITH ASPARAGUS

Ingredients:

- 4 salmon fillets
- 1 lb asparagus, trimmed
- 2 tbsp olive oil
- 2 cloves garlic, minced
- 1 lemon, sliced
- Salt and pepper to taste

Prep Time: 10 minutes
Cooking Time: 20 minutes
Servings: 4

Instructions:

1. Preheat oven to 400°F (200°C).
2. Place salmon fillets and asparagus on a baking sheet. Drizzle with olive oil and sprinkle with garlic, salt, and pepper.
3. Arrange lemon slices on top of the salmon.
4. Bake for 15-20 minutes, until salmon is cooked through and asparagus is tender.
5. Serve with a side of brown rice or quinoa.

4. TURKEY MEATBALLS WITH ZOODLES

Ingredients:

- 1 lb ground turkey
- 1/4 cup grated Parmesan cheese
- 1/4 cup breadcrumbs
- 1 egg
- 2 cloves garlic, minced
- 1 tsp dried oregano
- Salt and pepper to taste
- 2 medium zucchinis, spiralized into zoodles
- 1 cup marinara sauce

Prep Time: 15 minutes
Cooking Time: 20 minutes
Servings: 4

Instructions:

1. Preheat oven to 375°F (190°C).

2. In a bowl, mix ground turkey, Parmesan cheese, breadcrumbs, egg, garlic, oregano, salt, and pepper. Form into meatballs and place on a baking sheet.
3. Bake for 15-20 minutes or until meatballs are cooked through.
4. In a skillet, heat marinara sauce. Add zoodles and cook for 2-3 minutes until tender.
5. Serve meatballs over zoodles, topped with extra marinara sauce.

5. SHRIMP STIR-FRY WITH VEGETABLES

Ingredients:

- 1 lb shrimp, peeled and deveined
- 2 tbsp soy sauce
- 1 tbsp sesame oil
- 1 red bell pepper, sliced
- 1 yellow bell pepper, sliced
- 1 cup snap peas
- 1 carrot, julienned
- 2 cloves garlic, minced
- 1 tsp grated ginger

Prep Time: 10 minutes
Cooking Time: 10 minutes
Servings: 4

Instructions:

1. In a bowl, marinate shrimp with soy sauce and sesame oil for 10 minutes.
2. In a large skillet or wok, heat a small amount of oil. Add garlic and ginger, and sauté for 1 minute.
3. Add bell peppers, snap peas, and carrot, and stir-fry for 3-4 minutes.
4. Add shrimp and cook until pink and opaque, about 3-4 minutes.
5. Serve over brown rice or quinoa.

6. CHICKPEA AND SPINACH CURRY

Ingredients:

- 1 can (15 oz) chickpeas, rinsed and drained
- 1 onion, chopped
- 2 cloves garlic, minced
- 1 tbsp ginger, minced
- 1 can (14 oz) diced tomatoes
- 1 can (14 oz) coconut milk
- 2 cups spinach
- 2 tbsp curry powder
- 1 tbsp olive oil
- Salt and pepper to taste

Prep Time: 10 minutes
Cooking Time: 20 minutes
Servings: 4

Instructions:

1. In a large pot, heat olive oil over medium heat. Add onion, garlic, and ginger, and sauté until onion is translucent.
2. Add curry powder and cook for 1 minute.
3. Add chickpeas, diced tomatoes, and coconut milk. Bring to a simmer and cook for 10 minutes.
4. Stir in spinach and cook until wilted. Season with salt and pepper.
5. Serve over brown rice or quinoa.

CHAPTER 9

SPECIAL DIETS AND CONSIDERATIONS

In this chapter, we address the needs of individuals with specific dietary requirements, ensuring that everyone can enjoy delicious, healthy meals while effectively managing their weight. These recipes are designed to be inclusive, catering to gluten-free, dairy-free, vegetarian, and other dietary preferences and restrictions.

RECIPES

1. QUINOA AND BLACK BEAN STUFFED BELL PEPPERS (GLUTEN-FREE, VEGETARIAN)

Ingredients:

- 4 large bell peppers, tops cut off and seeds removed

- 1 cup quinoa, rinsed
- 2 cups vegetable broth
- 1 can (15 oz) black beans, drained and rinsed
- 1 cup corn kernels (fresh or frozen)
- 1 cup diced tomatoes
- 1 small onion, finely chopped
- 2 cloves garlic, minced
- 1 tsp cumin
- 1 tsp chili powder
- 1/2 tsp salt
- 1/4 cup chopped fresh cilantro

Prep Time: 15 minutes
Cooking Time: 45 minutes
Servings: 4

Instructions:

1. Preheat the oven to 375°F (190°C).
2. In a medium saucepan, combine quinoa and vegetable broth. Bring to a boil, then reduce to a simmer, cover, and cook for 15 minutes or until the quinoa is tender.
3. In a large bowl, mix cooked quinoa, black beans, corn, tomatoes, onion, garlic, cumin, chili powder, and salt.
4. Stuff each bell pepper with the quinoa mixture and place in a baking dish.
5. Cover with foil and bake for 30 minutes. Remove the foil and bake for an additional 10-15 minutes until the peppers are tender.
6. Garnish with chopped cilantro before serving.

2. CAULIFLOWER FRIED RICE (LOW-CARB, DAIRY-FREE)

Ingredients:

- 1 medium head of cauliflower, grated or processed into rice-sized pieces
- 2 tablespoons sesame oil
- 1 small onion, diced
- 2 cloves garlic, minced
- 1 cup frozen peas and carrots mix
- 2 eggs, beaten
- 3 tablespoons soy sauce (or tamari for gluten-free)
- 1/2 teaspoon ground ginger
- 3 green onions, sliced
- 1/4 cup chopped fresh cilantro

Prep Time: 10 minutes
Cooking Time: 15 minutes
Servings: 4

Instructions:

1. Heat sesame oil in a large skillet or wok over medium heat. Add onion and garlic, sauté until fragrant.
2. Add the peas and carrots mix, and cook until tender.
3. Push the vegetables to one side of the skillet and pour in the beaten eggs on the other side. Scramble

the eggs until fully cooked, then mix with the vegetables.
4. Add the cauliflower rice, soy sauce, and ground ginger. Stir-fry for about 5-7 minutes, until the cauliflower is tender but not mushy.
5. Stir in the green onions and cilantro before serving.

3. LEMON HERB BAKED SALMON (PALEO, DAIRY-FREE)

Ingredients:

- 4 salmon fillets
- 2 tablespoons olive oil
- 2 tablespoons lemon juice
- 1 tablespoon fresh dill, chopped
- 1 tablespoon fresh parsley, chopped
- 2 cloves garlic, minced
- Salt and pepper to taste
- Lemon slices for garnish

Prep Time: 10 minutes
Cooking Time: 20 minutes
Servings: 4

Instructions:

1. Preheat the oven to 400°F (200°C).
2. In a small bowl, mix olive oil, lemon juice, dill, parsley, garlic, salt, and pepper.

3. Place salmon fillets on a baking sheet lined with parchment paper. Brush the herb mixture over each fillet.
4. Garnish with lemon slices and bake for 15-20 minutes, or until the salmon flakes easily with a fork.

4. CHICKPEA AND SPINACH CURRY (VEGAN, GLUTEN-FREE)

Ingredients:

- 1 tablespoon coconut oil
- 1 large onion, diced
- 2 cloves garlic, minced
- 1 tablespoon ginger, minced
- 1 can (15 oz) diced tomatoes
- 1 can (15 oz) coconut milk
- 1 can (15 oz) chickpeas, drained and rinsed
- 4 cups fresh spinach
- 1 tablespoon curry powder
- 1 teaspoon ground cumin
- 1/2 teaspoon turmeric
- Salt and pepper to taste
- Cooked rice or quinoa for serving

Prep Time: 10 minutes
Cooking Time: 25 minutes
Servings: 4

Instructions:

1. Heat coconut oil in a large pot over medium heat. Add onion, garlic, and ginger, sauté until soft and fragrant.
2. Stir in curry powder, cumin, and turmeric, cooking for another minute.
3. Add diced tomatoes and coconut milk, bringing to a simmer.
4. Add chickpeas and spinach, cooking until the spinach is wilted and the chickpeas are heated through.
5. Season with salt and pepper. Serve over cooked rice or quinoa.

5. GRILLED CHICKEN WITH AVOCADO SALSA (KETO, DAIRY-FREE)

Ingredients:

- 4 boneless, skinless chicken breasts
- 2 tablespoons olive oil
- 1 teaspoon cumin
- 1 teaspoon paprika
- Salt and pepper to taste
- 2 avocados, diced
- 1 cup cherry tomatoes, halved
- 1/4 cup red onion, finely chopped
- 1 jalapeño, seeded and finely chopped

- 2 tablespoons lime juice
- 1/4 cup fresh cilantro, chopped

Prep Time: 15 minutes
Cooking Time: 15 minutes
Servings: 4

Instructions:

1. Preheat the grill to medium-high heat.
2. In a small bowl, mix olive oil, cumin, paprika, salt, and pepper. Brush the mixture over the chicken breasts.
3. Grill the chicken for 6-7 minutes on each side, or until fully cooked.
4. In a medium bowl, combine avocado, cherry tomatoes, red onion, jalapeño, lime juice, and cilantro. Season with salt and pepper.
5. Serve the grilled chicken topped with avocado salsa.

6. ZUCCHINI NOODLES WITH PESTO AND CHERRY TOMATOES (VEGETARIAN, GLUTEN-FREE)

Ingredients:

- 4 medium zucchinis, spiralized into noodles
- 2 cups cherry tomatoes, halved

- 1/4 cup pine nuts, toasted
- 1/2 cup fresh basil leaves
- 1/4 cup grated Parmesan cheese
- 1/4 cup olive oil
- 2 cloves garlic, minced
- Salt and pepper to taste

Prep Time: 15 minutes
Cooking Time: 5 minutes
Servings: 4

Instructions:

1. In a food processor, combine basil, Parmesan cheese, olive oil, garlic, salt, and pepper. Blend until smooth to make the pesto.
2. Heat a large skillet over medium heat. Add the zucchini noodles and cook for 2-3 minutes, until just tender.
3. Remove from heat and toss with pesto.
4. Add cherry tomatoes and toasted pine nuts. Serve immediately.

CHAPTER 10

MAINTAINING YOUR WEIGHT LOSS JOURNEY

Maintaining weight loss is often more challenging than losing weight in the first place. It requires a sustainable approach to eating and lifestyle changes that support your long-term health and well-being. This chapter focuses on strategies and recipes to help you keep the weight off and continue enjoying delicious, nutritious meals.

KEY STRATEGIES FOR MAINTAINING WEIGHT LOSS

1. **Balanced Eating:** Ensure each meal includes a balance of protein, healthy fats, and carbohydrates, focusing on whole foods.
2. **Portion Control:** Be mindful of portion sizes to avoid overeating.
3. **Regular Physical Activity:** Incorporate regular exercise into your routine, such as walking, jogging, or strength training.

4. **Stay Hydrated:** Drink plenty of water throughout the day.
5. **Mindful Eating:** Pay attention to your hunger and fullness cues, and avoid eating out of boredom or stress.
6. **Consistent Routine:** Stick to a consistent eating and exercise routine, even on weekends and holidays.
7. **Get Enough Sleep:** Aim for 7-9 hours of sleep per night to support overall health and weight maintenance.
8. **Seek Support:** Connect with friends, family, or a support group to stay motivated and accountable.

RECIPES

1. GRILLED CHICKEN AND QUINOA SALAD

Ingredients:

- 2 boneless, skinless chicken breasts
- 1 cup quinoa
- 2 cups water
- 1 cup cherry tomatoes, halved
- 1 cucumber, diced
- 1/4 cup red onion, finely chopped
- 2 cups mixed greens
- 2 tbsp olive oil

- 1 tbsp balsamic vinegar
- Salt and pepper to taste

Prep Time: 15 minutes
Cooking Time: 25 minutes
Servings: 4

Instructions:

1. Cook quinoa according to package instructions with 2 cups of water.
2. Season chicken breasts with salt and pepper. Grill over medium heat for 6-7 minutes per side or until fully cooked.
3. In a large bowl, combine cooked quinoa, cherry tomatoes, cucumber, red onion, and mixed greens.
4. Slice grilled chicken and place on top of the salad.
5. Drizzle with olive oil and balsamic vinegar. Toss to combine and serve.

2. BAKED SALMON WITH ASPARAGUS

Ingredients:

- 4 salmon fillets
- 1 bunch asparagus, trimmed
- 2 tbsp olive oil
- 1 lemon, sliced
- 2 garlic cloves, minced
- Salt and pepper to taste

Prep Time: 10 minutes
Cooking Time: 20 minutes
Servings: 4

Instructions:

1. Preheat oven to 400°F (200°C).
2. Place salmon fillets and asparagus on a baking sheet lined with parchment paper.
3. Drizzle with olive oil and sprinkle with minced garlic, salt, and pepper.
4. Top with lemon slices.
5. Bake for 15-20 minutes or until salmon is cooked through and asparagus is tender.
6. Serve immediately.

3. TURKEY AND VEGETABLE STIR-FRY

Ingredients:

- 1 lb ground turkey
- 2 cups broccoli florets
- 1 red bell pepper, sliced
- 1 yellow bell pepper, sliced
- 1 carrot, julienned
- 3 tbsp soy sauce (low sodium)
- 2 tbsp hoisin sauce
- 1 tbsp sesame oil
- 2 garlic cloves, minced
- 1 tsp ginger, grated

- 2 green onions, chopped

Prep Time: 15 minutes
Cooking Time: 15 minutes
Servings: 4

Instructions:

1. Heat sesame oil in a large skillet over medium heat.
2. Add ground turkey, garlic, and ginger. Cook until turkey is browned.
3. Add broccoli, bell peppers, and carrot. Stir-fry for 5-7 minutes until vegetables are tender-crisp.
4. Stir in soy sauce and hoisin sauce. Cook for an additional 2 minutes.
5. Garnish with chopped green onions and serve.

4. LENTIL AND SPINACH SOUP

Ingredients:

- 1 cup dried lentils, rinsed
- 6 cups vegetable broth
- 1 onion, diced
- 2 carrots, diced
- 2 celery stalks, diced
- 3 garlic cloves, minced
- 1 can (14.5 oz) diced tomatoes
- 2 cups fresh spinach, chopped
- 1 tsp cumin

- 1 tsp paprika
- Salt and pepper to taste
- 2 tbsp olive oil

Prep Time: 10 minutes
Cooking Time: 30 minutes
Servings: 4

Instructions:

1. Heat olive oil in a large pot over medium heat.
2. Add onion, carrots, celery, and garlic. Sauté until vegetables are tender.
3. Add lentils, vegetable broth, diced tomatoes, cumin, paprika, salt, and pepper. Bring to a boil.
4. Reduce heat and simmer for 25 minutes or until lentils are tender.
5. Stir in chopped spinach and cook for an additional 5 minutes.
6. Serve hot.

5. SHRIMP AND AVOCADO LETTUCE WRAPS

Ingredients:

- 1 lb shrimp, peeled and deveined
- 1 tbsp olive oil
- 1 tbsp lime juice
- 1 avocado, diced
- 1/4 cup red onion, finely chopped

- 1/4 cup cilantro, chopped
- 1 head butter lettuce, leaves separated
- Salt and pepper to taste

Prep Time: 10 minutes
Cooking Time: 10 minutes
Servings: 4

Instructions:

1. Heat olive oil in a skillet over medium heat.
2. Add shrimp, lime juice, salt, and pepper. Cook until shrimp are pink and opaque, about 3-4 minutes per side.
3. In a bowl, combine diced avocado, red onion, and cilantro.
4. Place shrimp and avocado mixture in the center of each lettuce leaf.
5. Serve immediately as wraps.

6. ZUCCHINI NOODLES WITH PESTO

Ingredients:

- 4 large zucchinis, spiralized
- 1 cup cherry tomatoes, halved
- 1/4 cup pine nuts
- 1/2 cup fresh basil leaves
- 1/4 cup grated Parmesan cheese
- 2 garlic cloves

- 1/4 cup olive oil
- Salt and pepper to taste

Prep Time: 15 minutes
Cooking Time: 5 minutes
Servings: 4

Instructions:

1. In a food processor, combine basil, Parmesan cheese, garlic, and pine nuts. Pulse until finely chopped.
2. With the processor running, slowly add olive oil until the mixture is smooth. Season with salt and pepper.
3. Heat a large skillet over medium heat. Add spiralized zucchini and cook for 2-3 minutes until just tender.
4. Remove from heat and toss with pesto sauce and cherry tomatoes.
5. Serve immediately.

CONCLUSION

Congratulations on taking a significant step towards achieving and maintaining a healthier lifestyle with "The Effective Weight Loss Cookbook." This journey is more than just a diet; it's a commitment to nourishing your body with wholesome, delicious foods that support your weight loss goals and overall well-being. Throughout this book, we've explored a wide range of recipes and strategies designed to make your weight loss journey enjoyable and sustainable.

KEY TAKEAWAYS

1. **Balanced Nutrition:** Embrace a diet rich in whole foods, including lean proteins, healthy fats, and complex carbohydrates. This balance helps keep you satisfied and energized throughout the day.
2. **Mindful Eating:** Pay attention to your body's hunger and fullness cues. Mindful eating helps you enjoy your meals more and prevents overeating.
3. **Portion Control:** Be mindful of portion sizes to avoid consuming excess calories. Use tools like measuring cups or food scales if necessary.
4. **Regular Physical Activity:** Incorporate exercise into your daily routine. Physical activity not only

aids in weight loss but also enhances your overall health and mood.
5. **Hydration:** Drink plenty of water to stay hydrated. Sometimes thirst is mistaken for hunger, leading to unnecessary snacking.
6. **Consistent Routine:** Establish a consistent eating and exercise routine. This helps create healthy habits that are easier to maintain in the long run.
7. **Support System:** Surround yourself with supportive friends, family, or join a community that shares your health goals. A strong support system can keep you motivated and accountable.
8. **Sustainable Changes:** Focus on making sustainable lifestyle changes rather than temporary fixes. Quick diets may provide short-term results, but lasting weight loss comes from consistent, healthy habits.

FINAL THOUGHTS

Remember, the journey to weight loss and maintenance is personal and unique to each individual. There will be ups and downs, but with determination and the right tools, you can achieve your goals. The recipes and strategies provided in this book are just the beginning. Continue exploring new foods, trying different exercises, and finding what works best for you.

Your health and well-being are worth the effort. By making informed choices and staying committed, you can enjoy a healthier, more fulfilling life. Keep experimenting in the kitchen, stay active, and never underestimate the power of a positive mindset.

Thank you for allowing "The Effective Weight Loss Cookbook" to be a part of your journey. Here's to your continued success, health, and happiness!

Wishing You All the Best

As you move forward, remember that each day is an opportunity to make choices that benefit your health. Celebrate your achievements, no matter how small, and keep pushing towards your goals. Your journey is unique, and every step you take is a step towards a healthier, happier you.

Printed in Great Britain
by Amazon